33 Prostate Cancer Meal Recipes That Will Help You Fight Cancer, Increase Your Energy, and Feel Better:

The Simple Solution to Your Cancer Problems

By

Joe Correa CSN

COPYRIGHT

ACKNOWLEDGEMENTS

This book is dedicated to my friends and family that have had mild or serious illnesses so that you may find a solution and make the necessary changes in your life.

33 Prostate Cancer Meal Recipes That Will Help You Fight Cancer, Increase Your Energy, and Feel Better:

The Simple Solution to Your Cancer Problems

By

Joe Correa CSN

CONTENTS

Copyright

Acknowledgements

About The Author

Introduction

33 Prostate Cancer Meal Recipes That Will Help You Fight Cancer, Increase Your Energy, and Feel Better: The Simple Solution to Your Cancer Problems

Additional Titles from This Author

ABOUT THE AUTHOR

After years of Research, I honestly believe in the positive effects that proper nutrition can have over the body and mind. My knowledge and experience has helped me live healthier throughout the years and which I have shared with family and friends. The more you know about eating and drinking healthier, the sooner you will want to change your life and eating habits.

Nutrition is a key part in the process of being healthy and living longer so get started today. The first step is the most important and the most significant.

INTRODUCTION

Cancer, in general, is a well-known disease that attacks many organs and other parts of our body, somehow it increases the abnormal growth of cells causing the spread of carcinoma in a process called metastases; although there are many treatments for cancer they are extremely invasive, and can many times kill good cells in the process. Prostate Cancer is a main concern for many men these days.

Preventing cancer is all about developing a style of life that involves a healthy diet and physical exercise. Being conscious about your food intake is the first step for a healthier life. To do that you should be aware of the qualities and properties of the foods you eat as well as the best way to cook them to get the maximum positive effects. The purpose of this book is to provide you with newer and better ways to nourish your body with non-processed foods, and in the process, changing your old eating habits for more promising ones.

Eating healthier can be delicious if you know what foods to combine and how. Eating smarter will drastically change how your body is able to use the vitamins and minerals you feed it to boost your immune system and prevent you from any kind of disease. Add these recipes to your day-to-day life to prevent and fight prostate cancer.

33 PROSTATE CANCER MEAL RECIPES THAT WILL HELP YOU FIGHT CANCER, INCREASE YOUR ENERGY, AND FEEL BETTER: THE SIMPLE SOLUTION TO YOUR CANCER PROBLEMS

1. FLAXSEED-CRANBERRY BREAD

This delicious bread recipe is more than an awesome and healthy treat, it is also perfect for a cancer preventive diet thanks to important compounds found in flaxseeds. Flaxseeds have an enormous amount of lignans which block and suppress carcinogenic cells, it is also rich in omega-3 fatty acids (as do walnuts) that are thought to protect against colon, heart and prostate cancer.

Ingredients:

- ¼ cup Lemon juice
- ¼ cup Canola oil
- ½ cup Honey
- 2 tsp Vanilla

- 1 cup Almond milk

- ½ cup Ground flaxseed

- 2 cups Whole wheat

- 2 tsp Baking powder

- 1 tsp Baking soda

- ¾ cup Dried or frozen cranberries

- ½ cups Walnuts, chopped

Instructions:

✓ Preheat oven to 350°F and oil a loaf pan;

✓ In a medium sized bowl whisk together lemon juice, oil, honey, vanilla and almond milk;

✓ Add the ground flaxseed and dry ingredients, stir until just combined;

✓ Toss the cranberries and walnuts and pour the batter into the prepared pan;

✓ Bake for 40 minutes, until golden brown;

✓ Let it cool before slicing.

2. GINGER MACKEREL & CUCUMBER SALAD

This amazing dish brings out the delicious taste and flavor of this ginger and cucumber combination. Ginger root is a powerful anti-inflammatory and anti-oxidant that acts by reducing the ability of tumors to grow. On the other hand, cucumber has lignans that have been shown to reduce the risk of uterine and prostate cancer.

Ingredients:

- 2 Mackerel fillets
- 1 Onion, chopped
- 1 Red pepper, chopped
- 1 lemon juice
- Fresh ginger, grated
- 1 garlic clove, minced
- 3 tbsp honey, separated 1-2
- 1 cucumber
- 2 tbsp dried wakame (seaweed)
- 4 tbsp Rice vinegar
- 1 tsp Sesame oil

- 1 tbsp Sesame seeds

- Salt and pepper to taste

Instructions:

✓ Rub the fish with salt and pepper;

✓ Prepare the marinade by mixing lemon juice, ginger and 1 tbsp honey, pour onto the fish and chill for about 30 minutes;

✓ Cut the cucumber into thin slices and sprinkle with salt, preserve for 10 minutes;

✓ Rehydrate the wakame by soaking in water as package instructions;

✓ Prepare the dressing mixing rice vinegar, sesame oil and remaining honey;

✓ Meanwhile, heat the grill and punt the fish skin side up on a baking sheet, grill for 5 minutes each side

✓ Wash and rinse the cucumber to remove the salt;

✓ Toss the cucumber and wakame together and sprinkle with sesame seeds;

✓ Serve the mackerel with the cucumber salad and spoon the dressing onto each serving.

3. STUFFED PEPPERS

With this dish you will enjoy the perks of organic bell peppers, turmeric, garlic, onions and tomatoes, all filth with vitamins and compounds that boost your system and protect your body. For example, turmeric stimulates the apoptosis in cancer and reduces tumor growth, and tomatoes are a high source of Lycopene that also aids preventing growth cell of prostate cancer.

Ingredients:

- 2 to 3 Colored bell peppers
- 1 cup Brown rice
- 1 tsp Cumin
- ½ tsp Turmeric
- 3 cups water
- Half Eggplant, chopped
- 1 Zucchini, chopped
- 1 Red Onion, diced
- 1 Garlic cloves, smashed
- 1 cup Natural tomato sauce

- 3 tbsp Olive oil

- Salt and pepper to taste

Instructions:

✓ Preheat the oven to 380°F;

✓ Prepare de peppers: cut side up and remove seeds, scrub them inside-out with salt and pepper;

✓ In a saucepan boiled the water, rice, cumin, turmeric and a dash of salt, for about 12 to 15 minutes;

✓ Wash, peel and cut the eggplant, zucchini and onions into dices;

✓ In an oiled saucepan stir fry the vegetables until softened;

✓ When rice is ready, add it in batches to the vegetables, mixing between batches;

✓ Add the tomato sauce and mix well;

✓ Spoon filing into the prepared peppers, cover them with foil and bake for 20 minutes;

✓ Remove the foil and bake for 3 to 5 more minutes.

4. RASPBERRY SALAD

This refreshing salad aims to care for your health, using the benefits of raspberries which contain ellagic acid, polyphenol and other compounds that promote the elimination of carcinogenic substances and inhibit angiogenesis.

Ingredients:

- 4 cups Romaine Lettuce, sliced
- 2 cups Cress
- 2 cups Radicchio
- 2 cups Raspberries
- ¼ cup Almonds, chopped
- 6 tbsp Natural Pomegranate juice
- 3 tbsp Olive oil
- 3 tbsp Apple vinegar
- 2 tbsp Honey
- Salt and pepper to taste

Instructions:

✓ Prepare the vinaigrette by mixing pomegranate juice, olive oil, apple vinegar, honey, salt and pepper, preserve;

✓ Wash and rinse the lettuce, cress and radicchio, cut roughly;

✓ In a big bowl put the green mixture and pour the vinaigrette on top and stir until combined;

✓ Sprinkle with almonds and serve.

5. FRUITY MORNING BOOSTER

Breakfast is the most important food of the day, this food will provide the energy to embrace your day full of energy while clean your body and revitalize your health. The incredible properties in these ingredients have shown to slow and prevent cancer development in color, liver, breast and prostate cells.

Ingredients:

- 1 Ripe bananas, smashed
- 1 cup Whole wheat
- ¾ cup Almond milk
- 1 egg, slightly beaten
- 1 tsp Baking powder
- 1 tsp Baking soda
- 1 tsp Salt
- 2 tsp Vanilla
- ¼ cup Walnuts, chopped
- Preferred jam, fresh fruits or maple syrup.
- 1 cup hot water

- 2 tsp Green tea

- 1 tsp Ginger, minced

- Half lemon juice

- Honey to taste

Instructions:

For the tea:

✓ Put the tea and ginger into the hot water and set aside while making the pancakes;

✓ Then add the lemon juice and honey.

For the pancakes:

✓ Blend together almond milk, egg, banana, wheat, baking powder, baking soda, salt and vanilla;

✓ Coated a skillet with cooking spray and heat over medium;

✓ Pour ¼ cup batter onto the pan and sprinkle with walnuts, cook 1 minute each side;

✓ Serve with preferred jam, fresh fruits or maple syrup.

6. DRIED TOMATOES FOCACCIA

This is a healthy meal option and a tasty treat. Keep enjoying the benefits of tomatoes, this time among whole-wheat, which is a great source of fiber. Dietary fiber is related with a lower risk some types of cancer, such as prostate, colon and colorectal cancer.

Ingredients:

- ¾ lukewarm water
- 2 tsp dry active yeast
- 1 tbsp honey
- 4 tbsp olive oil, divided
- 1 ½ cups whole wheat
- 1 tsp kosher salt
- 1 garlic clove, minced
- ½ cup dried tomatoes, chopped
- 1 tsp dried oregano

Instructions:

✓ Prepare a baking pan with baking spray;

✓ In a bowl combine water, yeast and honey, let it rest for 2 or 3 minutes;

✓ Add in the flour, garlic and oil, knead for 5 minutes;

✓ Spread the dough in the prepared pan and let it rise for 30 minutes;

✓ Once risen, preheat oven to 375°F;

✓ Sprinkle kosher salt, dried tomatoes and oregano over the dough and slightly press, drizzle with olive oil and bake for 10 minutes.

7. FUNFETTI CABBAGE SLAW

Red cabbage is rich flavonoids that prevent the growth of precancerous cells that can lead to colon, colorectal and prostate cancer. In addition, carrots are loaded with beta-carotene, which are known for preventing a wide range of cancers, including prostate cancer.

Ingredients:

- 2 tbsp apple vinegar
- 1 tsp honey
- 1 tsp Dijon mustard
- 1 tsp poppy seeds
- 1 tsp olive oil
- Salt and pepper to taste
- 1 cup green cabbage, thinly sliced
- 1 cup red cabbage, thinly sliced
- ½ cup carrots, shredded
- ¼ cup brazil nuts, chopped

Instructions:

✓ For the vinaigrette combine vinegar, honey, mustard, poppy seeds, olive oil, salt and pepper;

✓ Prepared the vegetables as described;

✓ Pour the vinaigrette onto the vegetables and toss;

✓ Sprinkle with brazil nuts and serve.

8. HEALTHY CHILI

This chili is full of ingredients that are packed with nutrients: turmeric, onions, carrots, peppers, garlic, beans, and tomatoes! Everything in this mouthwatering plate is designed to improve your health. Even the simplest thing like garlic has amazing benefits with many anti-cancer effects. This organosulfur compounds like allicin and alliin triggers cell death in prostate cancer.

Ingredients:

- 1 tbsp oil
- Half onion chopped
- 2 bay leaves
- 1 tsp cumin
- ½ tsp turmeric
- 2 stalks celery, chopped
- 1 carrot, peeled and chopped
- 2 bell peppers, chopped
- 1 chili pepper, chopped
- 2 garlic cloves, minced

- 1 cup kidney beans, cooked and drained

- 1 cup black beans, cooked and drained

- 2 tomatoes, cooked, peeled and chopped

- 1 cup kernel corn

- 2 tbsp chili powder

- Salt to taste

- Freshly ground black pepper

Instructions:

✓ Prepare the ingredients as described;

✓ Heat the oil in a sauce pan and toss onions, bay leaves, cumin, turmeric and salt;

✓ Add in celery, peppers and garlic, and simmer for 5 minutes;

✓ Mix the tomatoes, chili powder, black pepper and all beans, let it boiled then simmer for 20 minutes;

✓ Toss the corn and combine, cook for 5 more minutes;

✓ Serve hot.

9. MIGHTY BROCCOLI

Among the cruciferous, broccoli is well-known for preventing pre-cancerous cells from developing into malignant tumors; scientific studies demonstrated that it creates a strong defense against lung, prostate, breast, stomach, liver and ovarian cancer.

Ingredients:

- Olive oil
- 2 garlic clove, minced and divided
- 1 tbsp ginger, minced
- 4 cups Broccoli florets
- 1 Onion
- 2 tbsp honey
- 1 tbsp apple vinegar
- Kosher salt to taste
- Fresh ground black pepper to taste

Instructions:

✓ Preheat the oven to 400°F, prepare a baking pan coated with olive oil;

✓ Combine garlic, broccoli florets and salt, spread in the baking sheet and bake for 5 minutes

✓ Meanwhile, heat a skillet over medium with olive oil and sauté onions and a pinch of salt, until almost cooked;

✓ Add in garlic and ginger, stir over;

✓ Add honey and vinegar, low the heat;

✓ When ready, incorporate the broccoli and stir all together;

✓ Serve and enjoy.

10. VEGGIE LASAGNA

This veggie lasagna is the perfect replacement for processed pasta, and it also provides the benefits of mushrooms, which contain polysaccharides and Lentinant, both anti-carcinogenic compounds.

Ingredients:

- 1 tbsp olive oil
- 2 garlic cloves, minced
- 2 cups mushrooms
- 2 cups baby spinach
- 1 cup natural tomato sauce
- 2 to 3 zucchini, thinly sliced
- Salt and pepper to taste

Instructions:

✓ Preheat the oven to 375°F;

✓ Heat the oil in a skillet and add in garlic, mushroom, salt and pepper, cook for a couple minutes;

✓ Incorporate baby spinach and tomato sauce, cook for 3 or 4 minutes;

✓ In a baking dish spoon some sauce at the bottom and arrange zucchini slices on top, repeat until all ingredients have been used;

✓ Bake for 20 minutes;

✓ Let it cool for a few minutes and serve.

11. SAVORY PAPAYA SALAD

This exotic salad emphasizes the benefits of papayas, a rich fount of vitamin C and folic acid. This fruit has been shown to minimize absorption of cancer-causing nitrosamines from processed foods and prevent certain cancers, such as ovarian and prostate cancer.

Ingredients:

- 1 garlic cloves, minced
- Kosher salt to taste
- 2 tbsp Wine vinegar
- 2 tbsp honey
- 2 tsp sriracha sauce
- 1 firm papaya, seeded and diced
- 1 red onion, sliced
- 1 tsp paprika
- Fresh ground black pepper to taste

Instructions:

✓ Mix together papaya and onions

✓ In a medium bowl combine garlic, salt, vinegar, honey, sriracha sauce, paprika and ground pepper;

✓ Pour the mixture onto the papayas and onions and toss to incorporate;

✓ Serve and enjoy.

12. VEGGIE CURRY

Prepare to be pampered, with this veggie curry. You will absorb all the vitamins that you should to fight cancer. It will provide you with lots of lignans, flavonoids, beta-carotenes, lycopene, and more compounds that promise to take your health to another level and prevent you from getting a wide range of diseases.

Ingredients:

- Half onion, chopped
- 2 garlic cloves, smashed
- 1 tbsp ginger, grated
- ¼ dried tomatoes, chopped
- 1 tbsp olive oil
- 1 tsp cumin
- ½ tsp turmeric
- ½ tsp coriander
- 2 tbsp lentils
- 3 tbsp coconut milk
- 1 tbsp ground flaxseed

- ½ cup garbanzo beans, cooked and drained

- ½ cup pureed pumpkin

- Salt and pepper to taste

- Fresh coriander for sprinkle

Instructions:

✓ Blend together onion, garlic, ginger, pumpkin and tomatoes until it resembles a puree.

✓ Heat oil in a saucepan and add in cumin, turmeric and coriander, then incorporate the puree mixture and let it boil;

✓ Lower the heat and add lentils and coconut cream, simmer for 5 minutes;

✓ Stir garbanzo beans and flaxseed and cook for 3 to 5 more minutes;

✓ Serve and sprinkle with fresh coriander.

13. SAUCY SOUP

This saucy soup represents a new way to taste and harness the qualities of pumpkin and apples. On one hand, pumpkins are rich in carotenoids, lycopene and lutein, that increase the growth of immune cells and their capacity to attack tumor cells; on the other hand, apples are a good source of antioxidants and flavonoids.

Ingredients:

- 3 cups pureed pumpkin
- 2 large red apples
- 2 tbsp olive oil
- 2 cups chicken broth
- ½ tsp cinnamon
- Salt and pepper to taste
- ¼ chopped brazil nuts, for sprinkle

Instructions:

✓ In a skillet, heat oil and stir-fry diced apples with cinnamon, until apples start to caramelize;

✓ Incorporate pumpkin puree, then chicken broth, salt and pepper, cook for 7 minutes;

✓ Let it cool for a few minutes and blend together;

✓ Heat again if desired;

✓ Serve with Brazilian nuts sprinkled on top.

14.GREEN TEA AVOCADO ICE-CREAM

This ice-cream it's full of vitamins, starting with an avocado base that is highly rich in antioxidants, aiding your system to attack free radicals. This innovative way of eating avocado by mixing it with matcha (a Japanese green tea powder) is definitely an enhanced way to enjoy ice cream.

Ingredients:

- 2 avocados, peeled and frozen
- ½ cup almond milk
- ½ cup coconut milk
- 2 tbsp matcha powder
- ¼ cup dates, chopped
- Dash ground cardamom

Instructions:

✓ Blend together almond milk, coconut milk, dates, cardamom and matcha powder, *add 1 to 2 tbsp honey if desired;

✓ Gradually incorporate frozen avocado until reached a creamy texture;

✓ Serve immediately or freeze overnight.

15.MATCHA MUFFIN DELIGHT

We've been talking about the benefits of green tea, matcha is an incredible form of green tea powder. To enjoy its benefits let's use it in dishes for creating healthy desserts like this one. This Japanese green tea powder is the richest source of polyphenols and catechins that are known for inhibiting metastases. Also, dark chocolate chips bring out the real flavor while providing a great source of antioxidants.

Ingredients:

- 2/3 almond milk
- 2 tbsp cider vinegar
- 1 tbsp ground flaxseed
- 3 tbsp canola oil
- 1/3 honey
- Half banana, smashed
- 1 ½ whole wheat flour
- 2 tsp baking powder
- ½ tsp salt

- 2 tbsp matcha powder

- Dark chocolate chips *>70% cocoa

Instructions:

✓ Preheat the oven to 375°F and prepare a muffin pan;

✓ Combine almond milk, vinegar, and flaxseed, set aside for 5 minutes;

✓ Mix in oil, honey and banana;

✓ In a large bowl, combine flour, baking powder, salt and matcha powder;

✓ Pour liquid mixture into flour mixture and mix until almost combined (do not overmix);

✓ Add chocolate chips and slightly stir;

✓ Fill ¾ of the muffin pan with batter and bake for about 15 to 18 minutes.

16. GREEN STUFFED MUSHROOMS

In this plate we combined the powerful properties of mushrooms, garlic, spinach, bell pepper and onion, but also we incorporated seaweed (wakame), which contain molecules that slow cancer growth in breast, colon and prostate cancers.

Ingredients:

- 2 large Portobello mushrooms caps
- 2 tbsp olive oil, divided
- 1 garlic clove
- 1 cup baby spinach
- 1 cup green bell pepper, diced
- 1 small onion, diced
- ½ dried wakame
- 1 to 2 tbsp oyster sauce
- Salt and pepper to taste
- Sesame seeds for sprinkle

Instructions:

✓ Preheat oven to 400°F, slightly grease a baking pan;

✓ Rehydrate wakame as package instructions;

✓ In a large skillet heat the oil and stir fry bell pepper and onions until almost tender;

✓ Add spinach and garlic, sauté for a minute, and pour the oyster sauce, salt and pepper, cook for 3 to 4 more minutes;

✓ Remove from fire, stir rinsed wakame;

✓ Serve and sprinkle with sesame seeds.

17. SAUTEED SHRIMP & WHEAT-BERRY

Besides all the well-known benefits provided by broccoli, garlic, onion, scallions and endives, this recipe calls for wheat-berry, which contain wheat germ, thiamine, folate, zinc, and more compounds that ensure a balanced diet to prevent your system from any kind of disease.

Ingredients:

- 1 cup wheat berry
- 4 tbsp water
- 2 tbsp honey
- 2 tbsp rice vinegar
- 2 garlic clove, minced
- 2 cups broccoli florets
- 1 red onion, sliced
- 1 scallions, sliced
- 1 Belgian endive, sliced
- 2 cups raw shrimps
- 2 tbsp olive oil
- Salt and pepper to taste

Instructions:

✓ Cook wheat berry as package instructions say, drain and let it cool;

✓ Meanwhile, whisk together water, honey, vinegar and garlic;

✓ Heat a skillet oiled and sauté the drained wheat-berry over high heat, stir constantly until crispy, preserve in a bowl;

✓ In the same skillet, sauté broccoli for a couple of minutes, add in onions and endives, salt and pepper, cook for 5 minutes;

✓ Incorporate shrimps and cook, add the wet mixture and stir for 2 minutes;

✓ Return wheat berry and toss until everything's combine;

✓ Serve and sprinkle with scallions.

✓

18. MIX QUINOA SALAD

The meal has a lot of phytochemicals, lycopene, lignans and allicin that not only prevent your system from diseases, but help to fight any carcinogenic cells, inhibiting them from spreading around our body. This dish also uses quinoa to provide a great amount of soluble fibers.

Ingredients:

- ¾ cup uncooked quinoa
- 1 cup natural chicken broth
- ½ cup dried tomatoes, chopped
- 1 garlic clove, smashed
- 2 cups kale
- 2 cups red cabbage
- 1 avocado, peeled, pitted and chopped
- 1 tbsp olive oil
- 1 tbsp balsamic vinegar
- 3 tbsp brazil nuts, chopped
- Salt and pepper to taste

Instructions:

- ✓ Boil the broth and add in quinoa, salt and pepper, let it cook for 10 minutes, until the quinoa is tender and liquid is absorbed;

- ✓ In an oiled skillet quickly sauté garlic, kale, cabbage, salt and pepper, over high heat constantly stirring;

- ✓ Stir in quinoa and dried tomatoes, combine;

- ✓ Serve with avocados on top and drizzle with balsamic vinegar.

19. GREEN SOUP KICK

Fully charge your system with this green soup, with vegetables packed with beta-carotene, glutathione, vitamins, and many antioxidants that will increase the production of protective enzymes that inhibit angiogenesis. Also, brazil nuts contain a lot of selenium, which has been linked with prostate cancer treatments.

Ingredients:

- Half leek, sliced
- 1 garlic clove, minced
- 2 cups broccoli florets
- 2 cups asparagus, chopped
- 1 cup peas
- 5 cups natural vegetable or chicken broth
- 1 to 2 tsp sriracha sauce
- Half lemon juice
- Salt and fresh ground pepper to taste
- Chopped brazil nuts for sprinkle

Instructions:

✓ Heat an oiled skillet and sauté leeks for 5 minutes, toss garlic and cook for one more minute;

✓ Add broth, broccoli florets, asparagus and peas, let it simmer for 7 minutes;

✓ Blend the soup and season with sriracha, lemon, salt and pepper;

✓ Serve and sprinkle with chopped brazil nuts.

20. FRUITY BARS

Satisfy your cravings with these healthy fruity & nutty bars, rich in omega-3 fatty acids and many anti-carcinogenic agents found in peaches. On the other hand, pineapples are full of bromelain, an important component that fights cancer even better than the regular chemo drugs.

Ingredients:

- 1 ½ cup almond flour
- 1 ½ cup oat flour
- ½ cup honey
- 2 tbsp canola oil
- 3 cups peaches, chopped
- 1 cup nectarines, chopped
- 1 cups pineapples, chopped
- 1 cups cherries
- ½ cup orange juice
- ½ cup pomegranate juice
- 2 tsp granulated jelly

Instructions:

✓ Preheat the oven to 400°F and slightly grease a baking pan;

✓ Blend together almond flour, oat flour, honey and canola, until form clumps;

✓ Pour the mixture in to the baking pan and press down to form a layer, bake for 10 minutes or until golden brown;

✓ Meanwhile, prepare the filling heating an oiled saucepan to medium heat, stir in all the fruits and juice and simmer for 5 minutes;

✓ Mix the jelly with cold water;

✓ Remove the filling and cool for 5 minutes, incorporate hydrated jelly and stir until well combine;

✓ Pour the filling onto the baked crust and freeze over night;

✓ Cut the pie into bars and enjoy.

21. BEST-HEALTHY TOMATO SAUCE

We bring the ultimate healthy tomato sauce to boost your body with the goodness of lycopene in tomatoes. This recipe is packed with different vegetables that provide a high source of fiber. Mixing them together is the best way to get the most from all the nutrients in them.

Ingredients:

- 3 tbsp Olive oil
- 3 cloves Garlic, minced
- 1 large Onion, diced
- 1 large Carrots, diced
- 1 Green pepper, diced
- 1 Zucchini, diced
- 1 cup Natural Chicken broth
- 2 pounds Tomatoes
- 2 tsp Paprika
- 3 tsp dried Oregano
- 3 dried Bay leaves
- 3 dried Basil leaves

- Salt and pepper to taste

Instructions:

✓ In a large saucepan heat oil and add paprika, oregano bay and basil leaves, stir for less than a minute and incorporate carrots and peppers, cook for 3 minutes and toss onions, garlic and zucchini, salt and pepper, cook for 8 to 10 minutes, after this, using tongs remove bay and basil leaves;

✓ Meanwhile, in another saucepan bring water to boil and add the tomatoes for 5 to 7 minutes, until the peel starts to rip, remove from heat and add cold water. When cold, finish peeling the tomatoes and drain the remaining water;

✓ When peeled, blend the tomatoes with chicken broth and pour into the vegetables, let it simmer for 20 minutes, stirring occasionally;

✓ If desired, you can blend all the ingredients to have an homogenic sauce, and add one or two anchovies' fillets to make the perfect sauce for a pizza.

22.NO-KNEAD WHOLE WHEAT PIZZA DOUGH

Did you know there's a way to enjoy pizza and at the same time eat healthy? Because we all love to eat pizza, we want to show you a healthy pizza dough that can perfectly replace the processed pizza store. For enhanced taste and results, coat it with all natural tomato sauce, almond cheese (or other low fat cheese) and your favorite toppings.

Ingredients:

- 3 cups whole wheat flour
- 1 tbsp instant dry yeast
- 1 tsp kosher salt
- 1 cup lukewarm water
- 1 tbsp olive oil
- 1 tbsp honey

Instructions:

✓ In a large bowl combine dry ingredients;

✓ In a small bowl combine wet ingredients and pour it into the flour whilst stirring until incorporate and a shaggy dough forms;

✓ Transfer the dough into a clean and grease bowl and cover with plastic wrap, let it rest for 1 hour or until double it sizes;

✓ Gently deflate the dough using a wooden spoon, make two or three folders and let rest for 30 more minutes;

✓ When dough's ready, use a rolling pin to create a thin layer and cover with your favorites ingredients.

✓ Bake at 450°F for 10 to 13 minutes.

23.RASPBERRY CRUMBLES

This decadent dessert has an incredible taste perfect to satisfy any craving for sweets, and also provides a high amount of nutrients and compounds beneficial towards the prevention of cancer. Such is the case of the ellagic acid found in raspberries, which stimulates apoptosis, being a natural anti-carcinogenic and anti-mutagen fruit.

Ingredients:

- 2 cups raspberries
- 2 tbsp honey, divided
- 3 tbsp whole-wheat flour, divided
- 1 tbsp pomegranate juice
- ½ rolled oats
- ¼ cup chopped almonds
- ½ tsp cinnamon
- 1 tbsp canola oil

Instructions:

✓ Preheat oven to 400°F;

✓ Combine raspberries, 1 tbsp honey, pomegranate juice and 1 tbsp flour, divided among 4 ramekins;

✓ Combine oats, almonds, cinnamon, remaining honey and flour, add oil and stir until just combine. Sprinkle over the fruit mix;

✓ Bake for 20 minutes, let it cool for 15 minutes before serving.

24.MINI CALZONE

We want to teach you that been healthy doesn't mean you can't eat delicious food, so we bring this awesome mini calzone, a perfect treat for a family dinner while you stay on your nutritious diet.

Ingredients:

- 1 ball homemade "No-Knead Whole-Wheat Pizza Dough"
- 1 cup Tomato sauce
- ½ cup Almond cheese
- ½ cup Fresh basil
- 1 cup Baby spinach
- Half Red onion
- ¼ cup Black olives
- 1 tsp Dried Oregano
- 1 tsp Dried Garlic
- 1 tsp Dried Thyme
- 1 tsp Red pepper flakes
- ½ tsp Ground black pepper

- 2 tbsp Olive oil

- 1 egg

Instructions:

✓ Preheat oven to 400°F

✓ Cut the dough into 4 pieces, spread the pieces evenly in a floured surface to form 4 small pizzas;

✓ Toss all the filling ingredients together until combine;

✓ Spoon one or two tablespoon of filling mix on one half of each pizza and gently fold to form a half moon shape;

✓ Press the edges to seal;

✓ Coat with a beaten egg and sprinkle some kosher salt;

✓ Bake for 18 minutes.

25.TUNA HEALTHY-PATTIES

For this plate we are focusing on the goodness of omega-3 fatty acids contained in tuna fillets, the anti-inflammatory and antioxidant properties of ginger, as well as olive oil, that provides more antioxidants and vitamins for your daily life.

Ingredients:

- 2 Tuna fillets, skinless
- 1 tbsp Curry paste
- 1 tbsp fresh ginger, grated
- 1 tbsp fresh dill, minced
- 1 tbsp fresh coriander, minced
- 1 tsp olive oil
- Salt and pepper to taste

Ingredients:

- ✓ In a food processor, blend tuna fillets, curry paste, ginger, dill, coriander, salt and pepper;
- ✓ Pour the mix into a bowl and shape into a burger;

✓ In an oiled skillet, fry the burgers for 4 minutes each side.

✓ Serve with whole wheat bread and preferred salad.

26.SWEET & SPICY SALMON SUNSET

In this plate we combine sweetness and spiciness from mango and jalapeños, mangos are full of vitamins and beta-carotene compounds, while jalapeños are high in capsaicin that neutralize substance that might cause cancer.

Ingredients:

- 2 Salmon fillets
- 1 big mango, peeled and diced
- 1 red jalapeño, seeded and minced
- 1 fresh lemongrass, minced
- 1 tbsp rice vinegar
- 1 tbsp honey
- 2 tbsp olive oil, divided
- Salt and pepper to taste

Ingredients:

- ✓ Rub the fillets with salt and pepper;
- ✓ Combine mango, jalapeño, lemongrass, vinegar and honey;

✓ In a skillet heat 1 tablespoon of oil, place the salmon and cook for 3 minutes each side, set aside;

✓ In the same skillet heat the remaining oil and stir fry the mango mix for 3 or 4 minutes, add in the salmon and coat with juices and fruits;

✓ Remove from heat and serve;

27.FIG SALAD

Figs are awesome fruits for preventing and fighting cancer. Thanks to its derivatives of benzaldehyde, figs have been demonstrated to shrink tumors, and is also a great bacteria-killer.

Ingredients:

- 4 figs, chopped
- 4 cups Romaine lettuce, chopped
- ½ Basil leaves
- ¼ Pecans, chopped
- 3 tbsp Cider vinegar
- 2 tbsp Fig relish
- 1 tbsp Olive oil
- Salt and pepper to taste

Instructions:

- ✓ In a small bowl whisk together vinegar, relish, oil, salt and pepper;
- ✓ Toss the remaining ingredients in a large bowl;

✓ Pour dressing onto the green salad and combine;

✓ Serve with one piece of fig on top and sprinkle more chopped pecans.

28.COLORFUL SKEWERS

Skewers represent a fun way of cooking and eating, and in this case these colorful skewers are filled with vitamins and beta-carotene found in bell peppers. Also it provides the benefits of bromelain from the pineapple, as mentioned before, this potent compound fights cancer and is more effective than chemo drugs.

Ingredients:

- 1 Red pepper, chopped
- 1 Green pepper, chopped
- 1 Yellow pepper, chopped
- 1 Red onions, chopped
- 2 cups chopped Pineapples
- 2 tbsp Olive oil
- 1 Lemon juice
- 2 Garlic cloves, minced
- 1 tsp Paprika
- Salt and pepper to taste

Instructions:

✓ Prepare all ingredients as described and thread them into the skewers alternating the ingredients;

✓ Whisk together lemon, garlic, paprika, oil, salt and pepper;

✓ Coat the skewers with the marinade and let them marinate for 30 minutes;

✓ Grill for 10 to 15 minutes.

29.EASY GARLIC SOUP

As mentioned before, the anti-cancer benefits of garlic are many. Its immune-enhancing compounds aid the organism to fight and block carcinogenic cells, and studies have linked garlic to lower risk of stomach, colon and prostate cancer.

Ingredients:

- 6 tbsp Olive oil
- 1 garlic head
- 2 tbsp whole-wheat flour
- 4 cups natural chicken broth
- Dried Thyme
- Dried Oregano
- Dried Basil
- Salt and pepper to taste

Instructions:

✓ Cut garlic head in half -do not peel-;

✓ Heat an oiled saucepan to medium-low heat and place each half head flat, cook until garlic is soft and nicely browned, the peel will come out easily then;

✓ Remove from heat and smash the garlic with the flour combining well until a shaggy paste forms;

✓ Return to heat and add the hot broth, add thyme, oregano, basil, salt and pepper, cook until reached the desired consistency.

30.TUNA SALAD

Once again we want to use the benefits of tuna and its omega-3 fatty acids, but this time combining the properties of radish, which are high in anthocyanins which are powerful anti-cancer molecules that prevent carcinogenic cells from developing.

Ingredients:

- 2 tune fillet, stir-fry
- 1 Red pepper
- 1 Red onion
- 2 Tomatoes
- 3 cups romaine lettuce
- 2 cups radicchio
- 1 cup radish, sliced
- 3 tbsp Greek Yoghurt
- 1 Lemon juice
- 2 tbsp Olive oil
- ½ tsp Mustard seeds, grounded
- Salt and pepper to taste

Instructions:

✓ Whisk together yoghurt, oil, lemon, mustard seeds, salt and pepper;

✓ In a large bowl, combine peppers, onions, tomato, lettuce, radicchio and radish;

✓ Shred the tuna and stir it into the salad mixture;

✓ Drizzle with dressing and toss to incorporate.

31.BASIL ARUGULA PESTO

With this pesto you can create an awesome and healthy pizza or pasta, thanks to the essential oils in basil, which are part of the terpene family. They can promote apoptosis and reduce the spread of carcinogenic-cells.

Ingredients:

- 4 cups fresh basil
- 1 ½ cup fresh arugula
- 3 garlic cloves
- ½ brazil nuts
- Half lemon juice
- ¼ tsp lemon zest
- 4 tbsp chicken broth
- ¼ cup olive oil
- Salt and pepper to taste

Instructions:

✓ Pour all ingredients into a blender and blend until well mixed.

32. HEALTHY SANDWICH

Alkaline foods such as alfalfa and avocado keep blood ph in its ideal range, which is very important for the prevention and treatment of cancer.

Ingredients:

- 4 slices Whole-wheat nutty bread
- 200gr Smoked salmon
- 1 cup Alfalfa
- 1 cup Watercress
- 1 Avocado, smashed
- 3 tbsp Greek yoghurt
- 2 tbsp Olive oil
- Salt and pepper

Instructions:

✓ Smash avocado and mix in yoghurt, oil, salt and pepper;

✓ Coat bread slices with avocado mixture;

✓ Arrange salmon, alfalfa and watercress, and cover with bread.

33.JUICY CLEANSER

Fresh vegetable smoothies provide a valuable source of enzymes and antioxidant nutrients and are easily digestible. The well-known properties of pineapple, ginger, lemon and bee pollen makes this juice a perfect tonic for preventing cancer.

Ingredients:

- 1 cup Water
- Half Cucumber
- 1 cup chopped Pineapples
- 1 stalk Celery
- 1 Lemon, juiced
- 1 tsp Ginger, grated
- 1 tsp Bee pollen
- 1 tbsp Honey
- 2 tbsp chopped Almonds

Instructions:

✓ Rinse and peel fruits;

✓ Blend all ingredients together;

✓ Serve in a large glass and enjoy right away.

ADDITIONAL TITLES FROM THIS AUTHOR

70 Effective Meal Recipes to Prevent and Solve Being Overweight: Burn Fat Fast by Using Proper Dieting and Smart Nutrition

By

Joe Correa CSN

48 Acne Solving Meal Recipes: The Fast and Natural Path to Fixing Your Acne Problems in Less Than 10 Days!

By

Joe Correa CSN

41 Alzheimer's Preventing Meal Recipes: Reduce or Eliminate Your Alzheimer's Condition in 30 Days or Less!

By

Joe Correa CSN

70 Effective Breast Cancer Meal Recipes: Prevent and Fight Breast Cancer with Smart Nutrition and Powerful Foods

By

Joe Correa CSN

www.ingramcontent.com/pod-product-compliance
Lightning Source LLC
Chambersburg PA
CBHW072107040426
42334CB00042B/2575